Dash Diet Slow Cooker Cooking Guide

Stay Fit & Cook Quickly with This New Selection of Recipes

Carmela Rojas

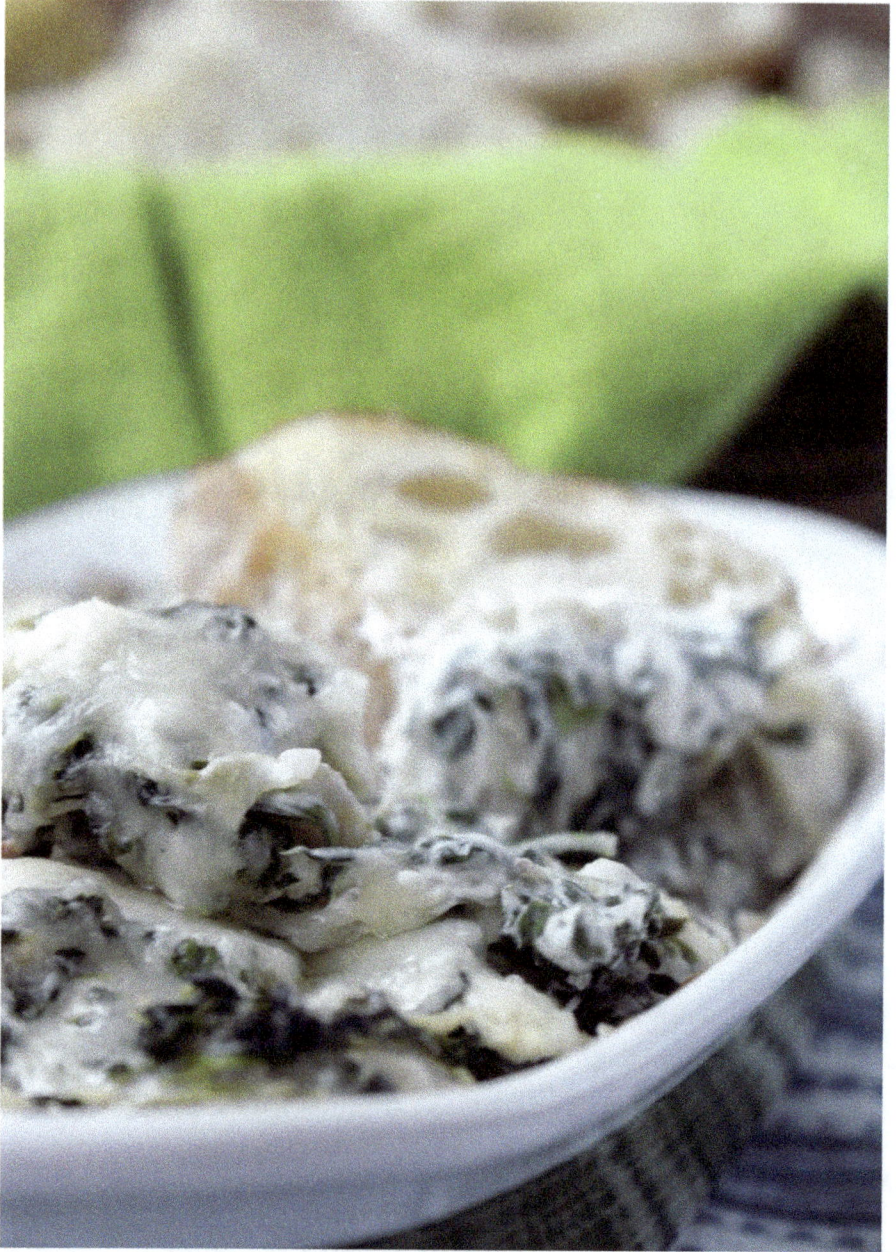

TABLE OF CONTENTS

Artichoke Spread

Servings: 8

Cooking Time: 30 Minutes

Ingredients:

- 4 cups spinach, chopped
- 2 cups artichoke hearts
- 1 cup white beans, already cooked
- 1 teaspoon thyme, chopped
- 2 garlic cloves, minced
- 1 tablespoon parsley, chopped
- 2 tablespoons low-fat parmesan, grated
- ½ cup low-fat sour cream
- Black pepper to the taste

Directions:

1. In your slow cooker, mix artichokes with spinach, black pepper, thyme, garlic, beans, parmesan, parsley and sour cream, stir, cover and cook on Low for 5 hours.
2. Transfer to your blender, pulse well divide into bowls and serve.

Nutrition Info:

Calories 145, Fat 3.5g, Cholesterol 6mg, Sodium 123mg, Carbohydrate 21.9g, Fiber 6.5g, Sugars 1.3g, Protein 8.5g, Potassium 714mg

Sausages And Shrimp Salad

Servings: 8

Cooking Time: 8 Hours

Ingredients:

- 4 cups low-sodium veggie stock
- 1 pound sausage, no extra salt added and sliced
- 2 pounds shrimp, deveined
- 2 tablespoons Italian seasoning
- 2 tablespoons parsley, chopped
- 4 tablespoons olive oil
- A pinch of black pepper

Directions:

1. In your slow cooker, mix stock with Italian seasoning, sausage, pepper, oil and shrimp, toss, cover, cook on Low for 8 hours, add parsley, toss, divide into small bowls and serve as an appetizer.

Nutrition Info:

Calories 406, Fat 26.1g, Cholesterol 289mg, Sodium 773mg, Carbohydrate 3.2g, Fiber 0g, Sugars 0.8g, Protein 36.9g, Potassium 366mg

Curry Dip

Servings: 10 Servings

Ingredients:

- ½ cup (58 g) shredded Cheddar cheese
- 8 ounces (225 g) fat-free cream cheese
- ¼ cup (60 ml) skim milk
- 1 teaspoon curry powder

Directions:

1. Mix ingredients together in slow cooker. Cover and cook on high 1 hour or until cheeses are melted. Stir.

Nutrition Info:

Per serving: 22 g water; 82 calories (68% from fat, 21% from protein, 10% from carb); 4 g protein; 6 g total fat; 4 g saturated fat; 2 g monounsaturated fat; 0 g polyunsaturated fat; 2 g carb; 0 g fiber; 0 g sugar; 75 mg phosphorus; 83 mg calcium; 0 mg iron; 112 mg sodium; 59 mg potassium; 235 IU vitamin A; 62 mg ATE vitamin E; 0 mg vitamin C; 20 mg cholesterol

Light Shrimp Salad

Servings: 8

Cooking Time: 5 Hours And 30 Minutes

Ingredients:

- 1 cup tomato, chopped
- ¼ pound shrimp, peeled, deveined and chopped
- 1 cup canned black beans, no-salt-added, drained and rinsed
- 1 cup cucumber, chopped
- 2 teaspoons cumin, ground
- 2 tablespoons olive oil
- ½ cup red onion, chopped
- Zest and juice of 2 limes
- Zest and juice of 2 lemons
- 2 tablespoons garlic, minced
- ¼ cup cilantro, chopped

Directions:

1. In a bowl, mix lime juice and lemon juice with shrimp and toss.

2. Grease the slow cooker with the oil, add black beans, tomato, onion, garlic and cumin, cover and cook on Low for 5 hours.

3. Add shrimp, cover, cook on Low for 30 minutes, more, transfer everything to a bowl, add cucumber and cilantro, toss, leave aside to cool down, divide between small bowls and serve as an appetizer.

Nutrition Info:

Calories 153, Fat 4.4g, Cholesterol 30mg, Sodium 40mg, Carbohydrate 21.4g, Fiber 15.2g, Sugars 2.3g, Protein 9.3g, Potassium 524mg

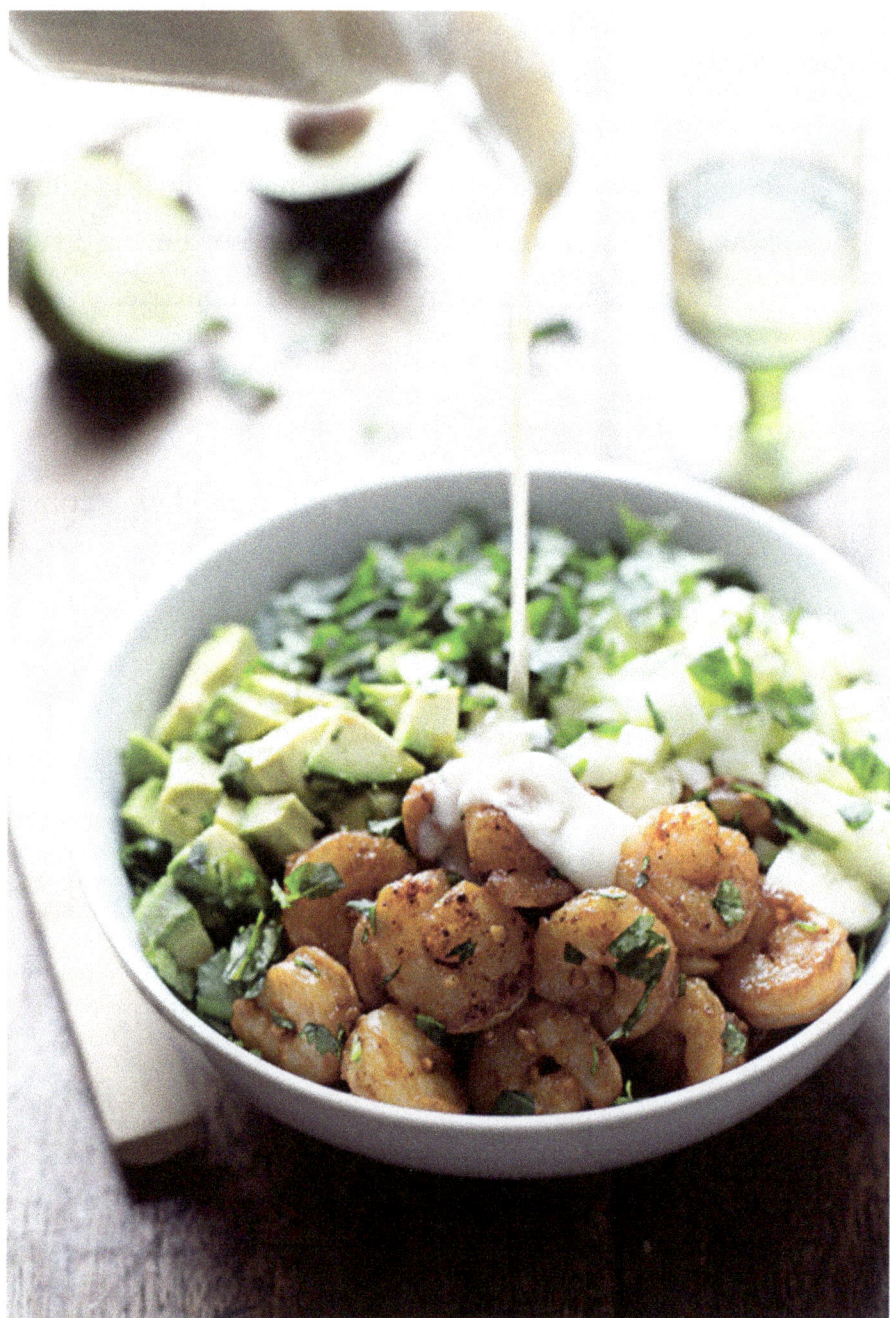

Hummus Spread

Servings: 10

Cooking Time: 3 Hours

Ingredients:

- 10 ounces hummus, no-salt-added
- 1 cup water
- 1 cup cashews
- 1 teaspoon apple cider vinegar
- ¼ teaspoon garlic powder
- ¼ teaspoon onion powder
- A pinch of black pepper

Directions:

1. In your slow cooker, mix water with cashews and pepper, stir, cover, cook on High for 3 hours, transfer to your blender, add hummus, garlic powder, onion powder and vinegar, pulse well, divide into bowls and serve.

Nutrition Info:

Calories 126, Fat 9.1g, Cholesterol 0mg, Sodium 110mg, Carbohydrate 8.6g, Fiber 2.1g, Sugars 0.7g, Protein 4.4g, Potassium 144mg

White Fish Salsa

Servings: 4

Cooking Time: 1 Hour And 30 Minutes

Ingredients:

- 15 ounces canned tomatoes, no-salt-added and chopped
- 1 pound cod fillets, skinless, boneless and cubed
- 1 red bell pepper, chopped
- 1 yellow onion, chopped
- 1 tablespoons rosemary, chopped
- ¼ cup low sodium veggie stock

Directions:

1. In your slow cooker, mix tomatoes with onion, bell pepper, rosemary and stock and stir.
2. Add fish, cover and cook on Low for 1 hour and 30 minutes.
3. Divide everything into bowls and serve warm as an appetizer.

Nutrition Info:

Calories 134, Fat 1.5g, Cholesterol 56mg, Sodium 103mg, Carbohydrate 9.7g, Fiber 2.6g, Sugars 5.5g, Protein 21.8g, Potassium 356mg

Pinto Bean Dip

Servings: 16 Servings

Ingredients:

- 2 pounds (910 g) lean ground beef
- 1 cup (160 g) chopped onion
- 2 cups (480 ml) refried beans
- 1½ cups (390 g) picante sauce
- Dash hot pepper sauce
- 1 teaspoon cumin
- ¼ teaspoon cayenne

Directions:

1. Combine ingredients in small slow cooker and heat until warm and cheese is melted, about 1 hour. Serve with corn chips.

Nutrition Info:

Per serving: 17 g water; 115 calories (21% from fat, 24% from protein, 55% from carb); 7 g protein; 3 g total fat; 2 g saturated fat; 1 g monounsaturated fat; 0 g polyunsaturated fat; 16 g carb; 4 g fiber; 1 g sugar; 138 mg phosphorus; 82 mg calcium; 1 mg iron; 75 mg sodium; 363 mg potassium; 119 IU vitamin A; 18 mg ATE vitamin E; 5 mg vitamin C; 7 mg cholesterol

Gourmet Mushrooms

Servings: 8 Servings

Ingredients:

- 1 pound (455 g) mushrooms
- ¼ cup (55 g) unsalted butter
- 1 cup (235 ml) low sodium chicken broth
- ¼ cup (60 ml) white wine
- 1 tablespoon (1.7 g) marjoram
- 1 tablespoon (3 g) chives

Directions:

1. Put cleaned mushrooms in slow cooker. Melt butter in a saucepan. Add remaining ingredients. Stir until thoroughly blended and then pour over mushrooms. Cook on high for 4 hours.

Nutrition Info:

Per serving: 89 g water; 75 calories (73% from fat, 13% from protein, 14% from carb); 2 g protein; 6 g total fat; 4 g saturated fat; 2 g monounsaturated fat; 0 g polyunsaturated fat; 3 g carb; 1 g fiber; 1 g sugar; 62 mg phosphorus; 10 mg calcium; 1 mg iron;

13 mg sodium; 217 mg potassium; 211 IU vitamin A; 48 mg ATE vitamin E; 2 mg vitamin C; 15 mg cholesterol

Meatballs In Apricot Sauce

Servings: 20

Cooking Time: 5 Hours

Ingredients:

- 12 ounces canned apricot preserves, unsweetened
- 2 pounds beef sausage, ground
- 2 eggs
- ½ cup yellow onion, chopped
- 2 tablespoons parsley, chopped
- ½ teaspoon garlic powder
- A pinch of black pepper

Directions:

1. In a bowl, mix beef sausage meat with eggs, onion, parsley, pepper and garlic powder, stir well and shape small meatballs out of this mix.
2. Put the meatballs in your slow cooker, add apricot preserves, toss, cover and cook on Low for 5 hours.
3. Arrange meatballs, sauce on a platter, and serve them.

Nutrition Info:

Calories 229, Fat 16.9g, Cholesterol 49mg, Sodium 378mg, Carbohydrate 12.6g, Fiber 0.1g, Sugars 7.6g, Protein 7g, Potassium 112mg

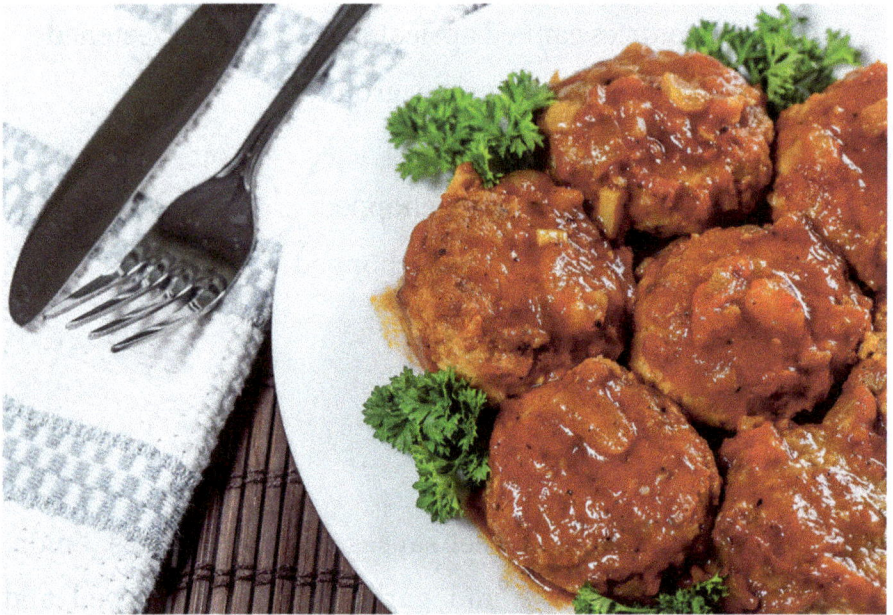

Pizza Dip

Servings: 12 Servings

Ingredients:

- 1 pound (455 g) extra-lean ground beef
- 3 cups (750 g) low-sodium spaghetti sauce
- 4 ounces (115 g) Cheddar, shredded
- 4 ounces (115 g) mozzarella, shredded
- 1 teaspoon oregano
- 1 teaspoon basil
- ½ teaspoon fennel seed

Directions:

1. Brown beef in a skillet over medium heat and crumble fine. Combine beef and remaining ingredients in slow cooker and cook on low for 2 to 3 hours.

Nutrition Info:

Per serving: 80 g water; 219 calories (58% from fat, 23% from protein, 19% from carb); 13 g protein; 14 g total fat; 6 g saturated fat; 6 g monounsaturated fat; 1 g polyunsaturated fat; 10 g carb; 2 g fiber; 7 g sugar; 169 mg phosphorus; 166 mg calcium; 1 mg iron; 161 mg sodium; 369 mg potassium; 535 IU vitamin A; 36 mg ATE vitamin E; 7 mg vitamin C; 42 mg cholesterol

Onion Chickpeas Dip

Servings: 12

Cooking Time: 2 Hours

Ingredients:

- 2 cups canned chickpeas, no-salt-added, drained and rinsed
- 1 cup red bell pepper, sliced
- 1 teaspoon onion powder
- 1 tablespoon lemon juice
- 1 teaspoon garlic powder
- 1 tablespoon olive oil
- 2 tablespoons white sesame seeds
- A pinch of cayenne pepper
- 1 and ¼ teaspoons cumin, ground

Directions:

1. In your slow cooker, mix red bell pepper with oil, sesame seeds, chickpeas, lemon juice, garlic and onion powder, cayenne pepper and cumin, cover and cook on High for 2 hours.
2. Transfer this mix to your blender, pulse well, divide into serving bowls and serve cold.

Nutrition Info:

Calories 143, Fat 3.8g, Cholesterol 0mg, Sodium 9mg, Carbohydrate 21.6g, Fiber 6g, Sugars 4.2g, Protein 6.8g, Potassium 321mg

Bourbon Hot Dogs

Servings: 24 Servings

Ingredients:

- 1 cup (240 g) no-salt-added ketchup
- 1 cup (225 g) brown sugar
- ½ cup (120 ml) bourbon
- 2 pounds (910 g) hot dogs, sliced

Directions:

1. Mix ketchup, brown sugar, and bourbon in slow cooker. Put hot dogs in and heat until hot dogs are cooked. Turn down to low and let them simmer in the sauce for at least an hour, then serve from the cooker.

Nutrition Info:

Per serving: 30 g water; 179 calories (61% from fat, 10% from protein, 29% from carb); 4 g protein; 11 g total fat; 5 g saturated fat; 6 g monounsaturated fat; 1 g polyunsaturated fat; 12 g carb; 0 g fiber; 12 g sugar; 58 mg phosphorus; 13 mg calcium; 1 mg iron; 393 mg sodium; 119 mg potassium; 93 IU vitamin A; 0 mg ATE vitamin E; 2 mg vitamin C; 21 mg cholesterol

Vegetable Dip

Servings: 7

Cooking Time: 5 Hours

Ingredients:

- 3 cups eggplant, cubed
- 10 ounces white mushrooms, chopped
- 6 garlic cloves, minced
- ½ cauliflower head, riced
- 54 ounces canned tomatoes, no-salt-added and crushed
- 2 tablespoons tomato paste, no-salt-added
- 2 tablespoons stevia
- 2 tablespoons balsamic vinegar
- 1 tablespoon basil, chopped
- 1 and ½ tablespoons oregano, chopped
- A pinch of black pepper

Directions:

1. In your slow cooker, mix cauliflower with tomatoes, mushrooms, eggplant, garlic, stevia, vinegar, tomato paste and pepper, stir, cover and cook on High for 5 hours.

2.   Add basil and oregano, stir, mash a bit with a potato masher, divide into bowls and serve as a dip.

Nutrition Info:

Calories 73, Fat 0.8g, Cholesterol 0mg, Sodium 25mg, Carbohydrate 18.9g, Fiber 5.4g, Sugars 8.6g, Protein 4.4g, Potassium 862mg

Tahini Dip

Servings: 4

Cooking Time: 3 Hours

Ingredients:

- ½ pound cauliflower florets
- 1 teaspoon avocado oil
- 1 tablespoon ginger, grated
- 1 cup coconut cream
- 3 garlic cloves, minced
- Black pepper to the taste
- 1 tablespoon basil, chopped
- 1 tablespoon tahini paste
- 1 tablespoon lime juice

Directions:

1. In your slow cooker, combine the cauliflower with the oil, ginger and the other ingredients, put the lid on and cook on Low for 3 hours.
2. Transfer to your blender, pulse well, divide into bowls and serve as a party dip.

Nutrition Info:

Calories 217, Fat 18.1g, Cholesterol 0mg, Sodium 311mg, Carbohydrate 13.3g, Fiber 3.5g, Sugars 5.7g, Protein 3.7g, Potassium 380mg

Queso Dip

Servings: 12 Servings

Ingredients:

- 1 cup (160 g) chopped onion
- 2 tablespoons (28 g) butter
- 4 ounces (115 g) jalapeños, chopped
- 2 cups (360 g) chopped tomatoes, undrained
- 4 ounces (115 g) pimientos, chopped and drained
- ¾ cup (90 g) grated Cheddar cheese

Directions:

1. Sauté onion in butter in medium saucepan. Combine jalapeños, tomatoes, pimientos, and cheese with onion and heat through; transfer to slow cooker and cook on low for 2 hours.

Nutrition Info: Per serving: 56 g water; 65 calories (64% from fat, 15% from protein, 20% from carb); 3 g protein; 5 g total fat; 3 g saturated fat; 1 g monounsaturated fat; 0 g polyunsaturated fat; 3 g carb; 1 g fiber; 1 g sugar; 55 mg phosphorus; 68 mg calcium; 0 mg iron; 106 mg sodium; 109 mg potassium; 560 IU vitamin A; 37 mg ATE vitamin E; 19 mg vitamin C; 14 mg cholesterol

Cheddar Dip

Servings: 6

Cooking Time: 2 Hours And 15 Minutes

Ingredients:

- 2 cups cauliflower rice
- 2 jalapenos, chopped
- ½ cup coconut cream
- 2 tablespoons chives, chopped
- ¼ cup low-fat cheddar cheese, grated
- A pinch of black pepper

Directions:

1. In your slow cooker, mix the jalapenos with the coconut cream, cauliflower, pepper, cheese and chives, stir, cover and cook on Low for 2 hours and 15 minutes.
2. Divide into bowls and serve.

Nutrition Info:

Calories 85, Fat 7g, Cholesterol 5mg, Sodium 72mg, Carbohydrate 3.7g, Fiber 0.6g, Sugars .2.2g, Protein 3g, Potassium 70mg

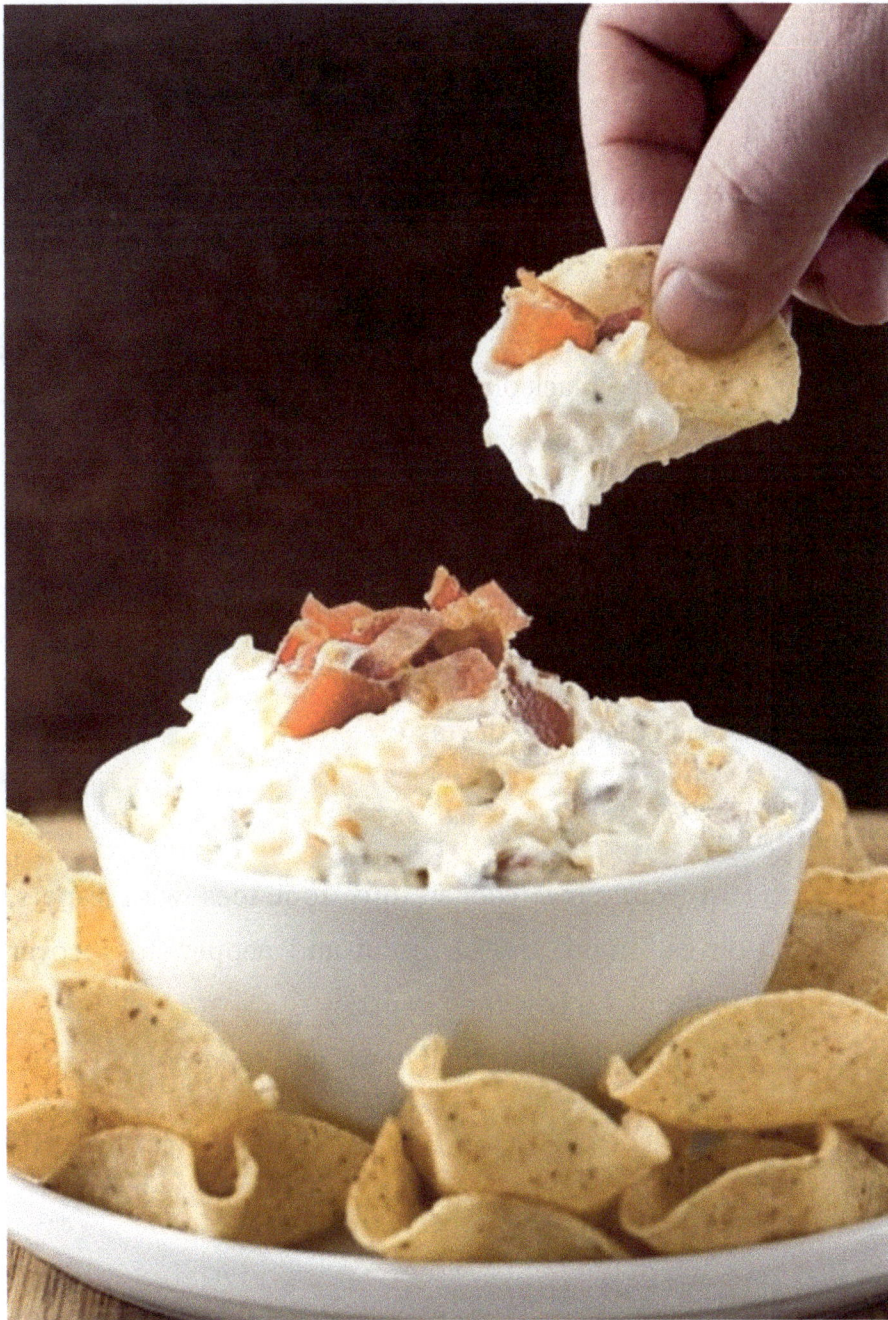

Balsamic Vinegar Salsa

Servings: 4

Cooking Time: 7 Hours

Ingredients:

- 8 ounces black olives, pitted and sliced
- 3 cups tomatoes, chopped
- 1 red onion, chopped
- 2 tablespoons mint, chopped
- 2 teaspoons capers, no-salt-added
- 2 teaspoons balsamic vinegar
- Black pepper to the taste

Directions:

1. In your slow cooker, mix tomatoes with capers, olives, onion, vinegar, mint and pepper, toss, cover and cook on Low for 7 hours.
2. Divide salsa into small bowls and serve cold.

Nutrition Info:

Calories 109, Fat 6.7g, Cholesterol 0mg, Sodium 601mg, Carbohydrate 12.6g, Fiber 4.3g, Sugars 5.2g, Protein 2.1g, Potassium 380mg

Dill And Scallions Salad

Servings: 4

Cooking Time: 2 Hours

Ingredients:

- 3 salmon fillets, skin on, boneless and cubed
- Zest of 1 lemon, grated
- 2 cups low-sodium chicken stock
- ¼ cup dill, chopped
- 4 scallions, chopped
- 3 black peppercorns
- ½ teaspoon fennel seeds
- 1 teaspoon white wine vinegar
- Black pepper to the taste

Directions:

1. In your slow cooker, mix lemon zest with scallions, peppercorns, fennel, pepper, vinegar, stock, dill and salmon, cover and cook on High for 2 hours.
2. Divide salmon and scallions salad into bowls and serve warm as an appetizer.

Nutrition Info:

Calories 200, Fat 8.7g, Cholesterol 59mg, Sodium 191mg, Carbohydrate 4.1g, Fiber 1.1g, Sugars 0.9g, Protein 27.4g, Potassium 662mg

Corn Salsa

Servings: 4

Cooking Time: 2 Hours

Ingredients:

- 1 pound green beans, trimmed and halved
- 1 cup corn
- 1 cup black olives, pitted and halved
- 2 tablespoons balsamic vinegar
- 1 cup cherry tomatoes, halved
- 2 tablespoons olive oil
- 2 garlic cloves, mince d
- 1 teaspoon rosemary, dried
- ½ cup low-sodium veggie stock

Directions:

1. In your slow cooker, combine the green beans with the corn, olives and the other ingredients, put the lid on and cook on High for 2 hours.
2. Divide into bowls and serve as an appetizer.

Nutrition Info:

Calories 182, Fat 11.3g, Cholesterol 0mg, Sodium 357mg, Carbohydrate 20.5g, Fiber 6.7g, Sugars 4.2g, Protein 4.1g, Potassium 465mg

Cumin And Avocado Salsa

Servings: 7

Cooking Time: 4 Hours

Ingredients:

- 1 cup canned black beans, no-salt-added, drained and rinsed
- 1 cup chunky salsa, salt-free
- 6 cups romaine lettuce, torn
- 1 tablespoon low sodium soy sauce
- ½ teaspoon cumin, ground
- ½ cup avocado, peeled, pitted and mashed

Directions:

1. In your slow cooker, mix the beans with salsa, cumin and soy sauce, stir, cover and cook on Low for 4 hours.
2. In a salad bowl, mix lettuce leaves with black beans mix and mashed avocado, toss, divide into small bowls and serve.

Nutrition Info:

Calories 134, Fat 2.6g, Cholesterol 0mg, Sodium 313mg, Carbohydrate 22.2g, Fiber 5.8g, Sugars 2.3g, Protein 7.1g, Potassium 646mg

Spinach Dip

Servings: 12 Servings

Ingredients:

- 8 ounces (225 g) cream cheese, cubed
- ¼ cup (60 ml) whipping cream
- 1 cup (190 g) frozen chopped spinach, thawed and squeezed dry
- 2 tablespoons (24 g) pimiento, diced
- 1 teaspoon Worcestershire sauce
- ¼ teaspoon garlic powder
- 2 tablespoons (10 g) grated Parmesan cheese
- 2 teaspoons finely chopped onion
- ¼ teaspoon thyme

Directions:

1. Combine cream cheese and cream in slow cooker. Cover and heat on low until cheese is melted, about 1 hour. Add remaining ingredients. Cover and heat on low 30 to 45 minutes longer.

Nutrition Info:

Per serving: 29 g water; 84 calories (80% from fat, 12% from protein, 8% from carb); 3 g protein; 8 g total fat; 5 g saturated fat; 2 g monounsaturated fat; 0 g polyunsaturated fat; 2 g carb; 1 g fiber; 0 g sugar; 38 mg phosphorus; 53 mg calcium; 1 mg iron; 92 mg sodium; 82 mg potassium; 2248 IU vitamin A; 76 mg ATE vitamin E; 3 mg vitamin C; 24 mg cholesterol

Stuffed Chicken With Spinach

Servings: 4

Cooking Time: 6 Hours

Ingredients:

- 4 chicken breasts, skinless and boneless
- 1 tablespoon olive oil
- 1 small yellow onion, chopped
- 2 chili peppers, chopped
- 1 red bell pepper, chopped
- 2 teaspoons garlic, minced
- 6 ounces spinach
- 1 tablespoon lemon juice
- 1 cup low-sodium veggie stock
- A pinch of black pepper
- A handful parsley, chopped

Directions:

1. Heat up a pan with the oil over medium-high heat, add bell pepper, chili peppers, onions, spinach, garlic, pepper and oregano, stir, cook for a couple of minutes and take off heat

2. Cut a pocket in each chicken breast, stuff with spinach mix, arrange in your slow cooker, add the stock, cover, cook on Low for 6 hours, arrange stuffed chicken on a platter, sprinkle parsley on top, drizzle the lemon juice and serve as an appetizer.

Nutrition Info:

Calories 342, Fat 14.7g, Cholesterol 130mg, Sodium 181mg, Carbohydrate 6.6g, Fiber 2g, Sugars 2.6g, Protein 44.7g, Potassium 702mg

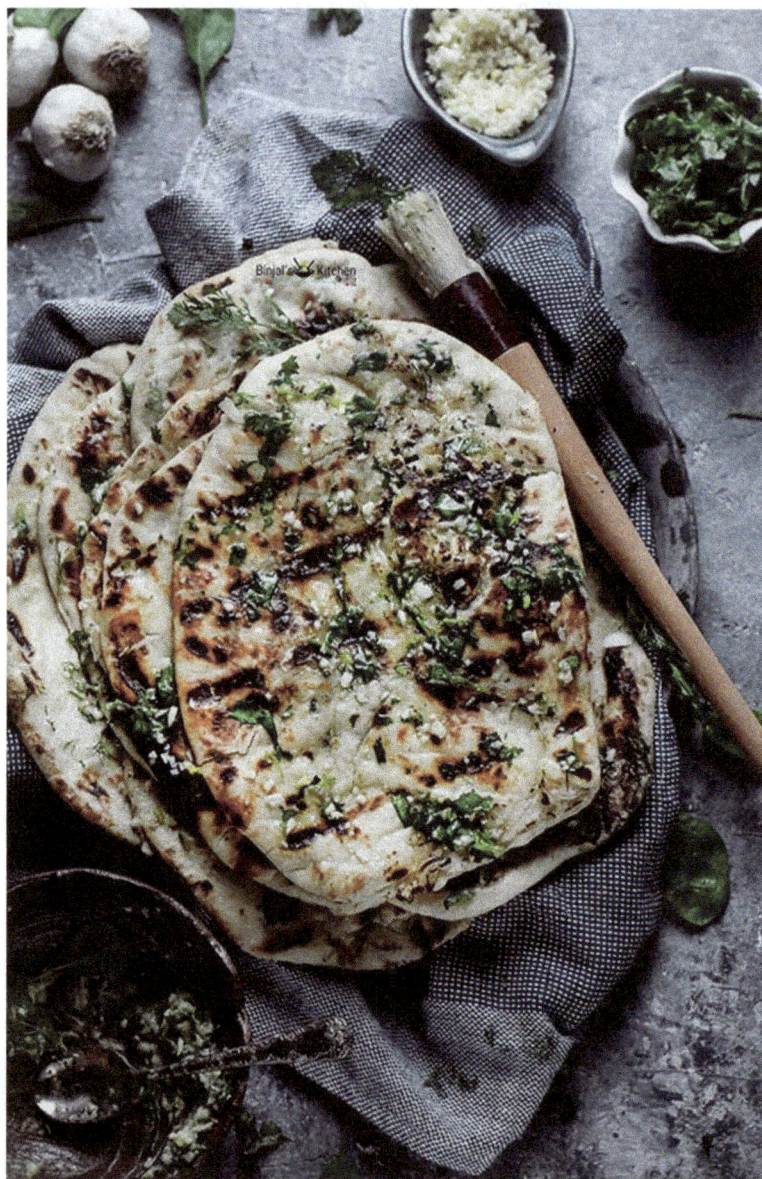

Seafood Dip

Servings: 4

Cooking Time: 1 Hour

Ingredients:

- 1 pound shrimp, peeled, deveined, cooked and chopped
- 1 cup low-fat cream cheese
- 1 cup coconut cream
- ½ cup low-fat cheddar, shredded
- 3 spring onions, chopped
- 1 tablespoon mustard
- 1 tablespoon lime juice
- 1 teaspoon turmeric powder

Directions:

1. In the slow cooker, combine the shrimp with the cream cheese and the other ingredients, put the lid on and cook on High for 1 hour.
2. Divide into small bowls and serve as a party dip.

Nutrition Info:

Calories 373, Fat 18.9g, Cholesterol 246mg, Sodium 691mg, Carbohydrate 11.4g, Fiber 2.2g, Sugars 2.9g, Protein 40g, Potassium 525mg

Cilantro Balls

Servings: 4

Cooking Time: 4 Hours

Ingredients:

- 14 ounces coconut milk
- 1 egg, whisked
- 1 and ½ pounds beef, minced
- 2 small yellow onions, chopped
- 3 tablespoons cilantro, chopped
- 2 tablespoons chili powder
- 1 teaspoon basil, dried
- 1 tablespoon green curry paste
- 1 tablespoon low sodium soy sauce
- Black pepper to the taste

Directions:

1. Put the meat in a bowl, add onion, egg, pepper and cilantro, stir well, shape medium-sized meatballs and place them in your slow cooker.
2. Add chili powder, soy sauce, milk, curry paste and basil, toss and cook on Low for 4 hours.

3. Arrange meatballs on a platter and serve them as an appetizer.

Nutrition Info:

Calories 606, Fat 37.1g, Cholesterol 193mg, Sodium 538mg, Carbohydrate 13.3g, Fiber 4.3g, Sugars 5.7g, Protein 56.4g, Potassium 1096mg

Shrimp Dip

Servings: 16 Servings

Ingredients:

- 16 ounces (455 g) fat free cream cheese
- 16 ounces (455 g) small frozen shrimp
- 1 cup (160 g) chopped onion
- ½ cup (90 g) chopped tomato

Directions:

1. Combine all ingredients in a slow cooker and cook slowly until cream cheese is melted and everything is cooked, about 2 hours. Keep warm in cooker. Serve with corn chips or toasted pita bread triangles.

Nutrition Info:

Per serving: 53 g water; 100 calories (50% from fat, 36% from protein, 14% from carb); 9 g protein; 5 g total fat; 3 g saturated fat; 1 g monounsaturated fat; 0 g polyunsaturated fat; 3 g carb; 0 g fiber; 1 g sugar; 104 mg phosphorus; 49 mg calcium; 1 mg iron; 127 mg sodium; 125 mg potassium; 283 IU vitamin A; 67 mg ATE vitamin E; 2 mg vitamin C; 59 mg cholesterol

Sweet Onion Dip

Servings: 12

Cooking Time: 5 Hours

Ingredients:

- 8 pounds tomatoes, peeled and chopped
- 6 ounces tomato paste, no-salt-added
- ¼ cup white vinegar
- 2 sweet onions, chopped
- 1 and ½ tablespoons Italian seasoning
- 2 tablespoons stevia
- ½ cup basil, chopped
- A pinch of black pepper

Directions:

1. In your slow cooker, mix the tomatoes with onions, tomato paste, vinegar, stevia, Italian seasoning, pepper and basil, stir, cover, cook on High for 5 hours, blend using an immersion blender, divide into bowls and serve as a dip.

Nutrition Info:

Calories 80, Fat 1.2g, Cholesterol 1mg, Sodium 30mg, Carbohydrate 18.5g, Fiber 4.6g, Sugars 10.6g, Protein 3.5g, Potassium 895mg

Sweet Salsa

Servings: 4

Cooking Time: 1 Hour

Ingredients:

- 3 mangoes, peeled and roughly cubed
- 1 cup black olives, pitted and halved
- 1 cup kalamata olives, pitted and halved
- 1 cup cherry tomatoes, cubed
- 1 cup corn
- Juice of ½ lemon
- 1 tablespoon olive oil
- 1 teaspoon garlic powder
- 1 tablespoon cilantro, chopped

Directions:

1. In the slow cooker, combine the mango with the olives, tomatoes and the other ingredients, put the lid on and cook on Low for 1 hour.
2. Divide into bowls and serve as an appetizer.

Nutrition Info:

Calories 429, Fat 23.3g, Cholesterol 0mg, Sodium 1258mg, Carbohydrate 57g, Fiber 6.8g, Sugars 37.1g, Protein 4.2g, Potassium450mg

Artichoke Dip

Servings: 8

Cooking Time: 2 Hours

Ingredients:

- 28 ounces canned artichokes, no-salt-added, drained and chopped
- 8 ounces coconut cream
- 10 ounces spinach
- 1 yellow onion, chopped
- ¾ cup coconut milk
- 2 garlic cloves, minced
- 3 tablespoons avocado mayonnaise
- 1 tablespoon red vinegar
- A pinch of black pepper

Directions:

1. In your slow cooker, mix artichokes with spinach, cream, onion, garlic, milk, mayo, vinegar and pepper, stir, cover, cook on Low for 2 hours, divide into bowls and serve as a snack.

Nutrition Info:

Calories 220, Fat 17.6g, Cholesterol 8mg, Sodium 173mg, Carbohydrate 15.6g, Fiber 7.1g, Sugars 2.7g, Protein 5.7g, Potassium 725mg

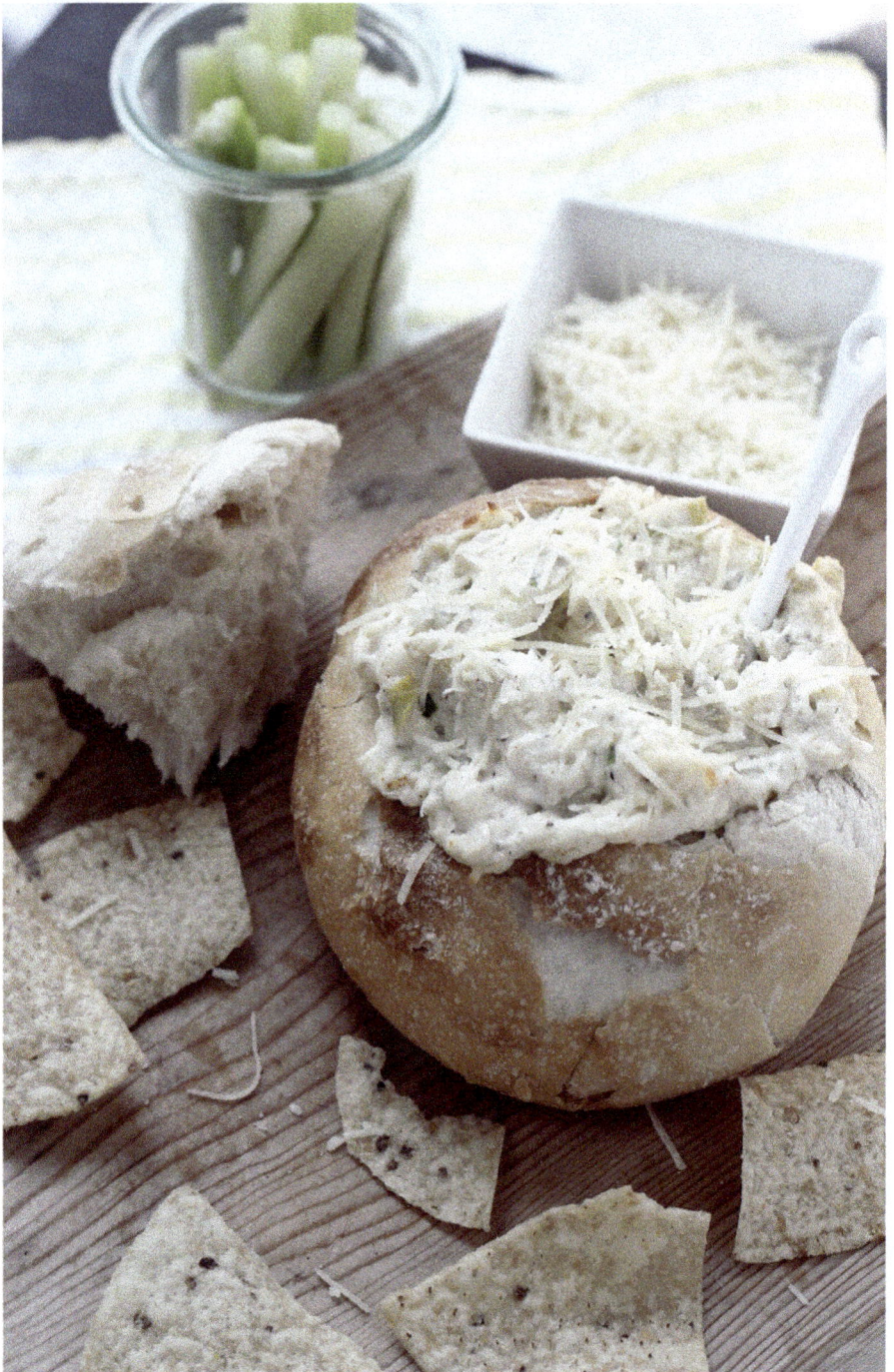

Cranberry Meatballs

Servings: 16 Servings

Ingredients:

- For Meatballs:
- 2 pounds (910 g) lean ground beef
- 1 cup (115 g) bread crumbs
- ½ cup (30 g) fresh parsley, chopped
- ½ cup (120 ml) egg substitute
- 1/3 cup (80 g) no-salt-added ketchup
- 3 tablespoons (30 g) minced onions
- 2 tablespoons (28 ml) low-sodium soy sauce
- ¼ teaspoon garlic powder
- ¼ teaspoon pepper
- For Sauce:
- 1 can (16 ounces, or 455 g) whole berry cranberry sauce
- 1½ cups (413 g) chili sauce
- 1 tablespoon (15 g) brown sugar
- 1 tablespoon (15 ml) lemon juice

Directions:

1. To make the meatballs: In a large bowl, combine ground beef, bread crumbs, parsley, egg substitute, ketchup, onion, soy sauce, garlic powder, and pepper. Mix well and form into small balls, from ½ inch (3 cm) to ¾ inch (2 cm) in diameter. Place in a casserole dish or baking pan. Heat oven to 300°F (150°C, or gas mark 2). Bake meatballs until nearly done, about 20 minutes.

2. To make the sauce: In a saucepan, combine cranberry sauce, chili sauce, brown sugar, and lemon juice. Cook, stirring, over medium heat until smooth. Transfer meatballs to slow cooker. Pour hot sauce over meatballs. Cook on low for 2 hours.

Nutrition Info:

Per serving: 88 g water; 229 calories (41% from fat, 23% from protein, 36% from carb); 13 g protein; 10 g total fat; 4 g saturated fat; 4 g monounsaturated fat; 1 g polyunsaturated fat; 20 g carb; 1 g fiber; 15 g sugar; 108 mg phosphorus; 31 mg calcium; 2 mg iron; 85 mg sodium; 248 mg potassium; 587 IU vitamin A; 0 mg ATE vitamin E; 8 mg vitamin C; 39 mg cholesterol

Beer Sausages

Servings: 16 Servings

Ingredients:

- 2 pounds (910 g) smoked sausage
- 1 cup (235 ml) beer
- ¼ cup (60 g) brown sugar
- 2 tablespoons (16 g) cornstarch
- ¼ cup (60 ml) vinegar
- ¼ cup (44 g) mustard
- 1 tablespoon (15 g) horseradish

Directions:

1. Cut sausage into ½-inch (3 cm) lengths. Boil them in beer for 10 minutes. Transfer to slow cooker. Mix brown sugar with cornstarch. Add to vinegar, mustard, and horseradish. Stir into slow cooker and cook on high for 2 hours.

Nutrition Info:

Per serving: 53 g water; 156 calories (60% from fat, 20% from protein, 19% from carb); 8 g protein; 10 g total fat; 4 g saturated fat; 5 g monounsaturated fat; 1 g polyunsaturated fat; 7 g carb; 0

g fiber; 3 g sugar; 4 mg phosphorus; 7 mg calcium; 1 mg iron; 390 mg sodium; 28 mg potassium; 3 IU vitamin A; 0 mg ATE vitamin E; 9 mg vitamin C; 40 mg cholesterol

French Style Salad

Servings: 6

Cooking Time: 9 Hours

Ingredients:

- 6 ounces canned tomato paste, no-salt-added
- 2 tomatoes, cut into medium wedges
- 2 yellow onions, chopped
- 1 eggplant, sliced
- 4 zucchinis, sliced
- 2 green bell peppers, cut into medium strips
- 2 garlic cloves, minced
- 2 tablespoons parsley, chopped
- 3 tablespoons olive oil
- 1 teaspoon oregano, dried
- 1 tablespoon basil, chopped
- A pinch of black pepper

Directions:

1. In your slow cooker, mix oil with onions, eggplant, zucchinis, garlic, bell peppers, tomato paste, tomatoes, basil, oregano and pepper, cover and cook on Low for 9 hours.

2. Add parsley, toss, divide into small bowls and serve warm as an appetizer.

Nutrition Info:

Calories 161, Fat 7.8g, Cholesterol 0mg, Sodium 48mg, Carbohydrate 22.8g, Fiber 7.3g, Sugars 12.7g, Protein 4.9g, Potassium 1047mg

Garlic And Beans Spread

Servings: 8

Cooking Time: 6 Hours

Ingredients:

- 15 ounces canned white beans, no-salt-added, drained and rinsed
- 8 garlic cloves, roasted
- 1 cup low-sodium veggie stock
- 2 tablespoons lemon juice
- 2 tablespoons olive oil

Directions:

1. In your blender, mix beans with oil, stock, garlic and lemon juice, cover, cook on Low for 6 hours, transfer to your blender, pulse well, divide into bowls and serve as a snack.

Nutrition Info:

Calories 214, Fat 4g, Cholesterol 0mg, Sodium 19mg, Carbohydrate 33.2g, Fiber 8.2g, Sugars 1.2g, Protein 12.9g, Potassium 971mg

Sweet and Sour Hot Dog Bites

Servings: 16 Servings

Ingredients:

- 1 cup (340 g) grape jelly
- ½ cup (88 g) mustard
- 1 pound (455 g) hot dogs, sliced
- 8 ounces (225 g) pineapple tidbits

Directions:

1. Microwave jelly until thin, about 30 seconds. Stir in mustard, hot dogs, and pineapple. Transfer to slow cooker and cook on low for 2 hours.

Nutrition Info:

Per serving: 34 g water; 160 calories (51% from fat, 9% from protein, 40% from carb); 4 g protein; 9 g total fat; 4 g saturated fat; 4 g monounsaturated fat; 0 g polyunsaturated fat; 16 g carb; 0 g fiber; 11 g sugar; 44 mg phosphorus; 14 mg calcium; 1 mg iron; 297 mg sodium; 84 mg potassium; 11 IU vitamin A; 0 mg ATE vitamin E; 3 mg vitamin C; 16 mg cholesterol

Taco Dip

Servings: 10 Servings

Ingredients:

- 16 ounces (455 g) fat-free cream cheese
- 1 teaspoon low-sodium onion soup mix
- 1 pound (455 g) extra-lean ground beef
- 2 teaspoons salt-free Mexican seasoning
- ½ cup (58 g) shredded Cheddar cheese
- ¼ cup (38 g) finely chopped green bell pepper

Directions:

1. Combine cream cheese and onion soup mix and spread in the bottom of slow cooker. In a skillet over medium-high heat, brown beef with Mexican seasoning. Place on top of cheese mixture. Sprinkle with Cheddar cheese, then green pepper. Cover and cook on low 2 to 3 hours.

Nutrition Info:

Per serving: 63 g water; 238 calories (69% from fat, 25% from protein, 6% from carb); 15 g protein; 18 g total fat; 10 g saturated fat; 6 g monounsaturated fat; 1 g polyunsaturated fat;

3 g carb; 0 g fiber; 0 g sugar; 165 mg phosphorus; 102 mg calcium; 2 mg iron; 205 mg sodium; 218 mg potassium; 388 IU vitamin A; 99 mg ATE vitamin E; 3 mg vitamin C; 64 mg cholesterol

Spicy Bean Dip

Servings: 32 Servings

Ingredients:

- 4 cups (952 g) refried beans
- 2 tablespoons (14 g) Salt-Free Mexican Seasoning
- ½ cup (80 g) chopped onion
- 2 cups (230 g) shredded Monterey Jack cheese
- 4 drops hot pepper sauce, or to taste
- Chopped jalapeños or mild chilies, to taste

Directions:

1. Place refried beans, Mexican seasoning, onion, cheese, and hot pepper sauce in the slow cooker; stir well to blend. Stir in chopped jalapeños or mild chilies. Cover and cook on low until cheese is melted, about 1 to 1½ hours; add a little water if mixture seems too thick. Serve from the slow cooker with French bread cubes, crackers, or chips.

Nutrition Info:

Per serving: 30 g water; 65 calories (40% from fat, 24% from protein, 36% from carb); 4 g protein; 3 g total fat; 2 g saturated fat; 1 g monounsaturated fat; 0 g polyunsaturated fat; 6 g carb; 2 g fiber; 0 g sugar; 64 mg phosphorus; 73 mg calcium; 1 mg iron; 219 mg sodium; 94 mg potassium; 190 IU vitamin A; 16 mg ATE vitamin E; 2 mg vitamin C; 10 mg cholesterol

Mushroom Dip

Servings: 6

Cooking Time: 4 Hours

Ingredients:

- 1 pound mushrooms, chopped
- 3 cups green bell peppers, chopped
- 28 ounces tomato sauce, no-salt-added
- 1 red onion, chopped
- 3 garlic cloves, minced
- ½ cup low-fat cheddar, grated
- Black pepper to the taste

Directions:

1. In your slow cooker, mix bell peppers with mushrooms, onion, garlic, tomato sauce, cheese and pepper, stir, cover, cook on Low for 4 hours, divide into bowls and serve.

Nutrition Info:

Calories 104, Fat 2g, Cholesterol 0mg, Sodium 737mg, Carbohydrate 17g, Fiber 4g, Sugars 11g, Protein 7.9g, Potassium 823mg

Mushroom Salsa With Pumpkin Seeds

Servings: 4

Cooking Time: 3 Hours

Ingredients:

- 1 pound white mushrooms, sliced
- 1 cup cherry tomatoes, halved
- 1 cup black olives, pitted and sliced
- 1 tablespoon olive oil
- Juice of 1 lime
- 2 tablespoons parsley, chopped
- 2 tablespoons pumpkin seeds
- 1 tablespoon basil, chopped
- 1 tablespoon balsamic vinegar

Directions:

1. In slow cooker, combine the mushrooms with the tomatoes, olives and the other ingredients, put the lid on and cook on Low for 3 hours.
2. Divide the salsa into bowls and serve as an appetizer.

Nutrition Info:

Calories 129, Fat 9.5g, Cholesterol 0mg, Sodium 304mg, Carbohydrate 9.4g, Fiber 3g, Sugars 3.4g, Protein 5.4g, Potassium 533mg

Parsley And Shrimps Cocktail

Servings: 4

Cooking Time: 2 Hours And 30 Minutes

Ingredients:

- 1 cup low-sodium chicken stock
- 40 shrimp, peeled and deveined
- 2 tablespoons olive oil
- 2 teaspoons garlic, minced
- 2 teaspoons parsley, chopped

Directions:

1. In your slow cooker, mix stock with oil, parsley, garlic and shrimp, toss, cover and cook on Low for 2 hours and 30 minutes.
2. Divide into bowls and serve as an appetizer.

Nutrition Info:

Calories 325, Fat 10.7g, Cholesterol 463mg, Sodium 571mg, Carbohydrate 3.8g, Fiber 0.1g, Sugars 0g, Protein 50.5g, Potassium 382mg

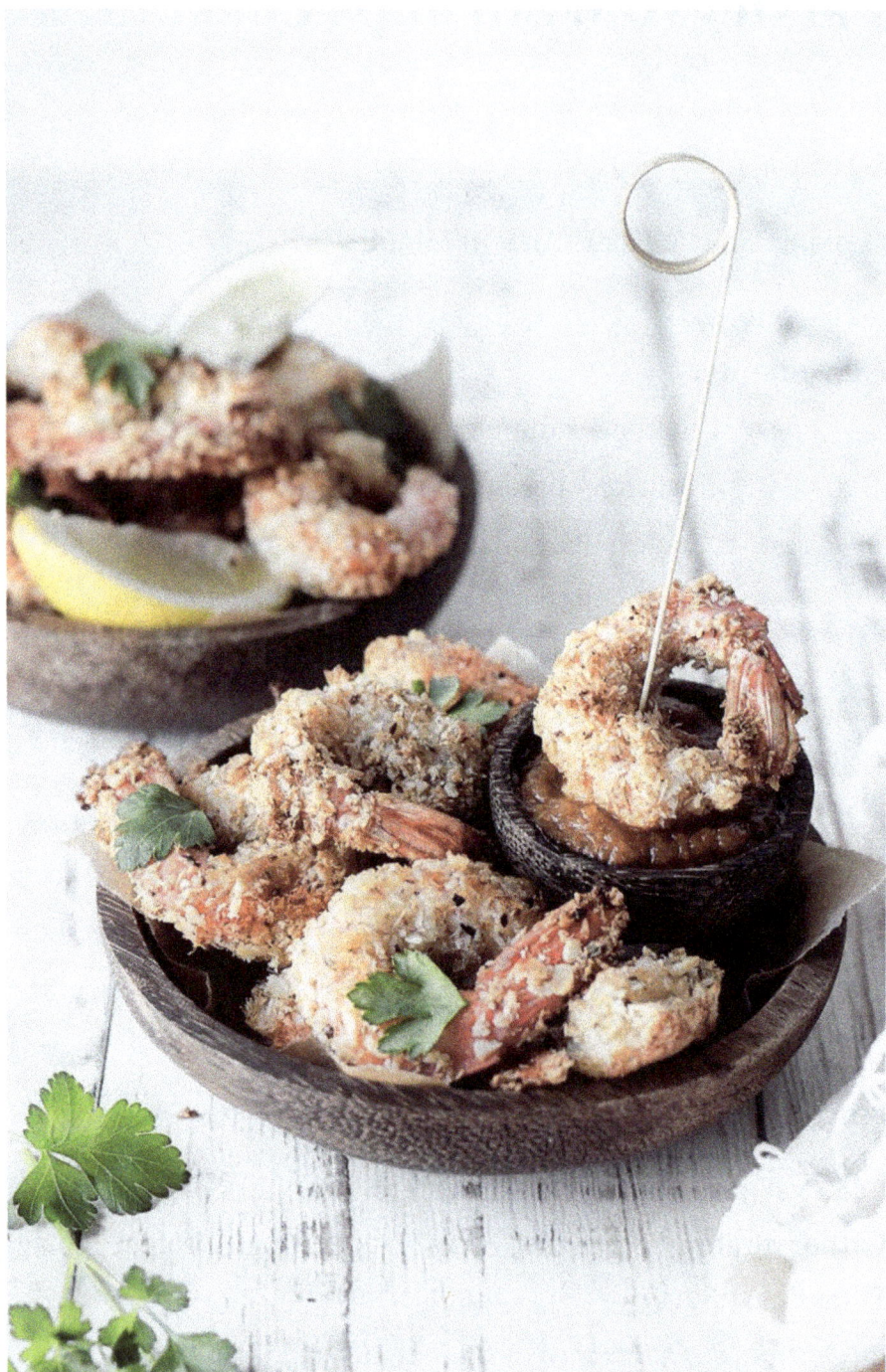

Salsa Cheese Dip

Servings: 24 Servings

Ingredients:

- 1 pound (455 g) Cheddar cheese, shredded
- 3 ounces (85 g) cottage cheese
- 4 ounces (115 g) canned green chilies
- 1½ cups (390 g) salsa

Directions:

1. Heat all ingredients in slow cooker. Cook on low until cheese melts and flavors are well mixed, about 2 hours.

Nutrition Info:

Per serving: 27 g water; 84 calories (67% from fat, 26% from protein, 7% from carb); 6 g protein; 6 g total fat; 4 g saturated fat; 2 g monounsaturated fat; 0 g polyunsaturated fat; 1 g carb; 0 g fiber; 1 g sugar; 105 mg phosphorus; 143 mg calcium; 0 mg iron; 169 mg sodium; 67 mg potassium; 238 IU vitamin A; 49 mg ATE vitamin E; 2 mg vitamin C; 20 mg cholesterol

Cumin Hummus

Servings: 6

Cooking Time: 5 Hours

Ingredients:

- 1 cup chickpeas, soaked overnight and drained
- 2 garlic cloves
- ¾ cup green onions, chopped
- 1 tablespoon olive oil
- 2 tablespoons sherry vinegar
- 3 cups water
- 1 teaspoon cumin, ground

Directions:

1. Put the water in your slow cooker, add chickpeas and garlic, cover and cook on Low for 5 hours.
2. Drain chickpeas, transfer them to your blender, add ½ cup of the cooking liquid, green onions, vinegar, oil, cilantro and cumin, blend well, divide into bowls and serve.

Nutrition Info:

Calories 150, Fat 4.5g, Cholesterol 0mg, Sodium 15mg, Carbohydrate 22.3g, Fiber 6.2g, Sugars 3.9g, Protein 6.8g, Potassium 338mg

Tuna Noodle Casserole

Servings: 6 Servings

Ingredients:

- 10 ounces (280 g) low-sodium cream of mushroom soup
- 1/3 cup (80 ml) low-sodium chicken broth
- 2/3 cup (160 ml) skim milk
- 2 tablespoons (2.6 g) dried parsley
- 10 ounces (280 g) frozen no-salt-added peas
- 14 ounces (390 g) tuna, well drained
- 10 ounces (280 g) egg noodles, cooked until just tender
- 3 tablespoons (21 g) bread crumbs

Directions:

1. Spray slow cooker with nonstick cooking spray. In a large bowl, combine soup, chicken broth, milk, parsley, peas, and tuna. Fold in the cooked noodles. Pour mixture into prepared slow cooker. Top with bread crumbs. Cover and cook on low for 5 to 6 hours.

Nutrition Info:

Per serving: 199 g water; 231 calories (14% from fat, 38% from protein, 49% from carb); 22 g protein; 4 g total fat; 1 g saturated fat; 1 g monounsaturated fat; 1 g polyunsaturated fat; 28 g carb; 5 g fiber; 3 g sugar; 278 mg phosphorus; 75 mg calcium; 2 mg iron; 273 mg sodium; 467 mg potassium; 1196 IU vitamin A; 22 mg ATE vitamin E; 7 mg vitamin C; 30 mg cholesterol

Tuna Stuffed Peppers

Servings: 4 Servings

Ingredients:

- 2 cups (475 ml) low-sodium tomato juice
- 1 can (6 ounces, or 170 g) no-salt-added tomato paste
- 14 ounces (390 g) tuna, drained and rinsed
- 2 tablespoons (30 g) dried minced onion
- ¼ teaspoon garlic powder
- 4 green bell peppers, tops removed and seeded

Directions:

1. Mix tomato juice and tomato paste, reserving 1 cup (235 ml). Mix remaining tomato mixture with tuna, minced onion, and garlic powder. Fill peppers equally with mixture. Place upright in slow cooker. Pour the reserved 1 cup (235 ml) tomato mixture over peppers. Cover and cook on low 8 to 9 hours or until peppers are done.

Nutrition Info:

Per serving: 359 g water; 222 calories (14% from fat, 48% from protein, 39% from carb); 28 g protein; 3 g total fat; 1 g saturated fat; 1 g monounsaturated fat; 1 g polyunsaturated fat; 22 g carb; 5 g fiber; 14 g sugar; 311 mg phosphorus; 63 mg calcium; 3 mg iron; 108 mg sodium; 1248 mg potassium; 1766 IU vitamin A; 6 mg ATE vitamin E; 153 mg vitamin C; 42 mg cholesterol

Tuna Vegetable Casserole

Servings: 6 Servings

Ingredients:

- 16 ounces (455 g) water-packed tuna
- 20 ounces (560 g) low-sodium cream of mushroom soup
- 1 cup (235 ml) milk
- 2 tablespoons (2.6 g) dried parsley
- 10 ounces (280 g) frozen mixed vegetables, thawed
- 10 ounces (280 g) egg noodles, cooked and drained
- ¼ cup (30 g) sliced almonds, toasted

Directions:

1. Combine tuna, soup, milk, parsley, and vegetables. Fold in noodles. Spray slow cooker with nonstick cooking spray and pour tuna mixture in. Top with almonds. Cover and cook on low 7 to 9 hours or on high 3 to 4 hours.

Nutrition Info:

Per serving: 248 g water; 286 calories (23% from fat, 34% from protein, 43% from carb); 24 g protein; 7 g total fat; 1 g saturated fat; 3 g monounsaturated fat; 2 g polyunsaturated fat; 30 g carb; 6 g fiber; 6 g sugar; 343 mg phosphorus; 101 mg calcium; 2 mg iron; 104 mg sodium; 739 mg potassium; 2259 IU vitamin A; 31 mg ATE vitamin E; 3 mg vitamin C; 35 mg cholesterol

Dijon Fish

Servings: 4 Servings

Ingredients:

- 1¼ pounds (570 g) orange roughy fillets
- 2 tablespoons (22 g) Dijon mustard
- 3 tablespoons (42 g) unsalted butter, melted
- 1 teaspoon Worcestershire sauce
- 1 tablespoon (15 ml) lemon juice

Directions:

1. Cut fillets to fit in slow cooker. In a bowl, mix remaining ingredients together. Pour sauce over fish. Cover and cook on low 3 hours or until fish flakes easily but is not dry or overcooked.

Nutrition Info:

Per serving: 119 g water; 191 calories (47% from fat, 50% from protein, 2% from carb); 24 g protein; 10 g total fat; 6 g saturated fat; 3 g monounsaturated fat; 1 g polyunsaturated fat; 1 g carb; 0 g fiber; 0 g sugar; 164 mg phosphorus; 20 mg calcium; 2 mg iron; 201 mg sodium; 264 mg potassium; 373 IU vitamin A; 101 mg ATE vitamin E; 4 mg vitamin C; 108 mg cholesterol

Fish Pie

Servings: 4 Servings

Ingredients:

- 1 pound (455 g) haddock, or other firm white fish
- 10 ounces (280 g) frozen corn
- 10 ounces (280 g) no-salt-added frozen peas
- ½ cup (115 g) fat-free cream cheese
- 2/3 cup (160 ml) skim milk
- ¼ cup (30 g) bread crumbs
- ½ cup (58 g) shredded Cheddar cheese

Directions:

1. Cut fish into bite-size pieces. Combine with corn and peas and place into slow cooker. Stir cream cheese and milk until well blended and pour over fish mixture. Cover and cook on high until fish is done, about 2 hours. Preheat oven to 400°F (200°C, or gas mark 6). Combine bread crumbs and cheese and sprinkle over fish. Remove liner from slow cooker and bake until cheese melts and topping begins to brown, about 10 minutes.

Nutrition Info:

Per serving: 263 g water; 394 calories (29% from fat, 37% from protein, 33% from carb); 37 g protein; 13 g total fat; 7 g saturated fat; 4 g monounsaturated fat; 1 g polyunsaturated fat; 33 g carb; 6 g fiber; 6 g sugar; 516 mg phosphorus; 279 mg calcium; 4 mg iron; 354 mg sodium; 776 mg potassium; 2153 IU vitamin A; 141 mg ATE vitamin E; 12 mg vitamin C; 100 mg cholesterol

Salmon Loaf

Servings: 6 Servings

Ingredients:

- 16 ounces (455 g) canned salmon
- ½ cup (120 ml) egg substitute
- 1½ cups (175 g) bread crumbs
- ¼ cup (40 g) finely chopped onion
- 2 tablespoons (28 g) unsalted butter, melted
- 1 tablespoon (4 g) fresh parsley
- 1 tablespoon (15 ml) lemon juice
- Dash cayenne

Directions:

1. Drain salmon; reserve juices. If necessary, add water to juices to make ¼ cup (60 ml) liquid. Combine liquid with remaining ingredients except the salmon. Flake salmon; stir into mixture. Shape into round loaf slightly smaller in diameter than slow cooker. Line cooker with foil to come up 2 or 3 inches (5 or 7.5 cm) on sides. Place loaf on foil, not touching sides. Cover and cook on low for 5 hours.

Nutrition Info:

Per serving: 82 g water; 268 calories (35% from fat, 34% from protein, 31% from carb); 22 g protein; 10 g total fat; 4 g saturated fat; 3 g monounsaturated fat; 2 g polyunsaturated fat; 20 g carb; 1 g fiber; 2 g sugar; 341 mg phosphorus; 252 mg calcium; 2 mg iron; 95 mg sodium; 366 mg potassium; 293 IU vitamin A; 45 mg ATE vitamin E; 2 mg vitamin C; 40 mg cholesterol

Seafood Jambalaya

Servings: 4 Servings

Ingredients:

- 4 slices low sodium bacon, chopped
- 1 cup (160 g) chopped onion
- ¾ cup (75 g) sliced celery
- ½ teaspoon minced garlic
- ½ teaspoon cayenne
- 1 teaspoon oregano
- ½ teaspoon thyme
- 2 cups (360 g) no-salt-added diced tomatoes
- 3 cups (705 ml) vegetable broth
- 1½ cups (278 g) uncooked long-grain rice
- 8 ounces (225 g) catfish, cut in 1-inch (2.5 cm) cubes
- 8 ounces (225 g) shrimp, peeled

Directions:

1. Cook the bacon, onion, celery, and garlic in a skillet until bacon is crisp and vegetables are softened. Transfer to slow cooker. Add remaining ingredients except fish and shrimp, cover, and cook on low until rice is tender, about 4 hours. Turn to high, add fish

and shrimp, cover, and cook until fish flakes easily, about 30 minutes to 1 hour.

Nutrition Info:

Per serving: 472 g water; 379 calories (32% from fat, 30% from protein, 38% from carb); 28 g protein; 13 g total fat; 3 g saturated fat; 6 g monounsaturated fat; 3 g polyunsaturated fat; 36 g carb; 3 g fiber; 5 g sugar; 381 mg phosphorus; 126 mg calcium; 4 mg iron; 312 mg sodium; 757 mg potassium; 476 IU vitamin A; 40 mg ATE vitamin E; 20 mg vitamin C; 122 mg cholesterol

Salmon Casserole

Servings: 6 Servings

Ingredients:

- 4 medium potatoes, peeled and sliced
- 3 tablespoons (24 g) flour
- 16 ounces (455 g) salmon, drained and flaked
- ½ cup (80 g) chopped onion
- 10 ounces (280 g) low-sodium cream of mushroom soup
- ¼ cup (60 ml) water
- Dash nutmeg

Directions:

1. Spray slow cooker with nonstick cooking spray. Place half of the potatoes in slow cooker. Sprinkle with half of the flour. Cover with half the flaked salmon and then sprinkle with half the onion. Repeat layers. Combine soup and water; pour over top of potato and salmon mixture. Sprinkle with just a dash of nutmeg. Cover and cook on low for 7 to 9 hours or until potatoes are tender.

Nutrition Info:

Per serving: 316 g water; 323 calories (15% from fat, 27% from protein, 58% from carb); 22 g protein; 5 g total fat; 1 g saturated fat; 2 g monounsaturated fat; 2 g polyunsaturated fat; 47 g carb; 5 g fiber; 4 g sugar; 450 mg phosphorus; 223 mg calcium; 3 mg iron; 253 mg sodium; 1547 mg potassium; 67 IU vitamin A; 15 mg ATE vitamin E; 22 mg vitamin C; 31 mg cholesterol

Lemon Catfish

Servings: 4 Servings

Ingredients:

- 1½ pounds (680 g) catfish fillets
- ½ cup (80 g) chopped onion
- 1 tablespoon (1.3 g) parsley
- 4 teaspoons (8 g) grated lemon rind

Directions:

1. Spray slow cooker with nonstick cooking spray. Place fish in cooker. Put onion, parsley, and lemon rind over fish. Cover and cook on low for 1½ hours.

Nutrition Info:

Per serving: 148 g water; 239 calories (50% from fat, 46% from protein, 4% from carb); 27 g protein; 13 g total fat; 3 g saturated fat; 6 g monounsaturated fat; 3 g polyunsaturated fat; 2 g carb; 1 g fiber; 1 g sugar; 350 mg phosphorus; 24 mg calcium; 1 mg iron; 92 mg sodium; 546 mg potassium; 165 IU vitamin A; 26 mg ATE vitamin E; 6 mg vitamin C; 80 mg cholesterol

Corn Chowder With Crab

Servings: 4 Servings

Ingredients:

- 6 slices low-sodium bacon, diced
- ¼ cup (40 g) chopped onion
- 2 potatoes, peeled and diced
- 1 pound (455 g) frozen corn
- 1 tablespoon (13 g) sugar
- 1 teaspoon Worcestershire sauce
- ¼ teaspoon pepper
- ½ cup (120 ml) water
- 1 cup (235 ml) skim milk
- 6 ounces (170 g) crab meat

Directions:

1. In skillet, brown bacon until crisp. Remove bacon, reserving drippings. Add onions and potatoes to skillet and sauté for 5 minutes. Drain. Combine all ingredients in slow cooker except milk and crab meat. Mix well. Cover and cook on low 6 to 7 hours. Stir in milk and crab during the last 30 minutes of cooking.

Nutrition Info:

Per serving: 336 g water; 364 calories (15% from fat, 22% from protein, 62% from carb); 21 g protein; 6 g total fat; 2 g saturated fat; 3 g monounsaturated fat; 1 g polyunsaturated fat; 59 g carb; 6 g fiber; 9 g sugar; 412 mg phosphorus; 152 mg calcium; 2 mg iron; 280 mg sodium; 1351 mg potassium; 155 IU vitamin A; 40 mg ATE vitamin E; 25 mg vitamin C; 48 mg cholesterol

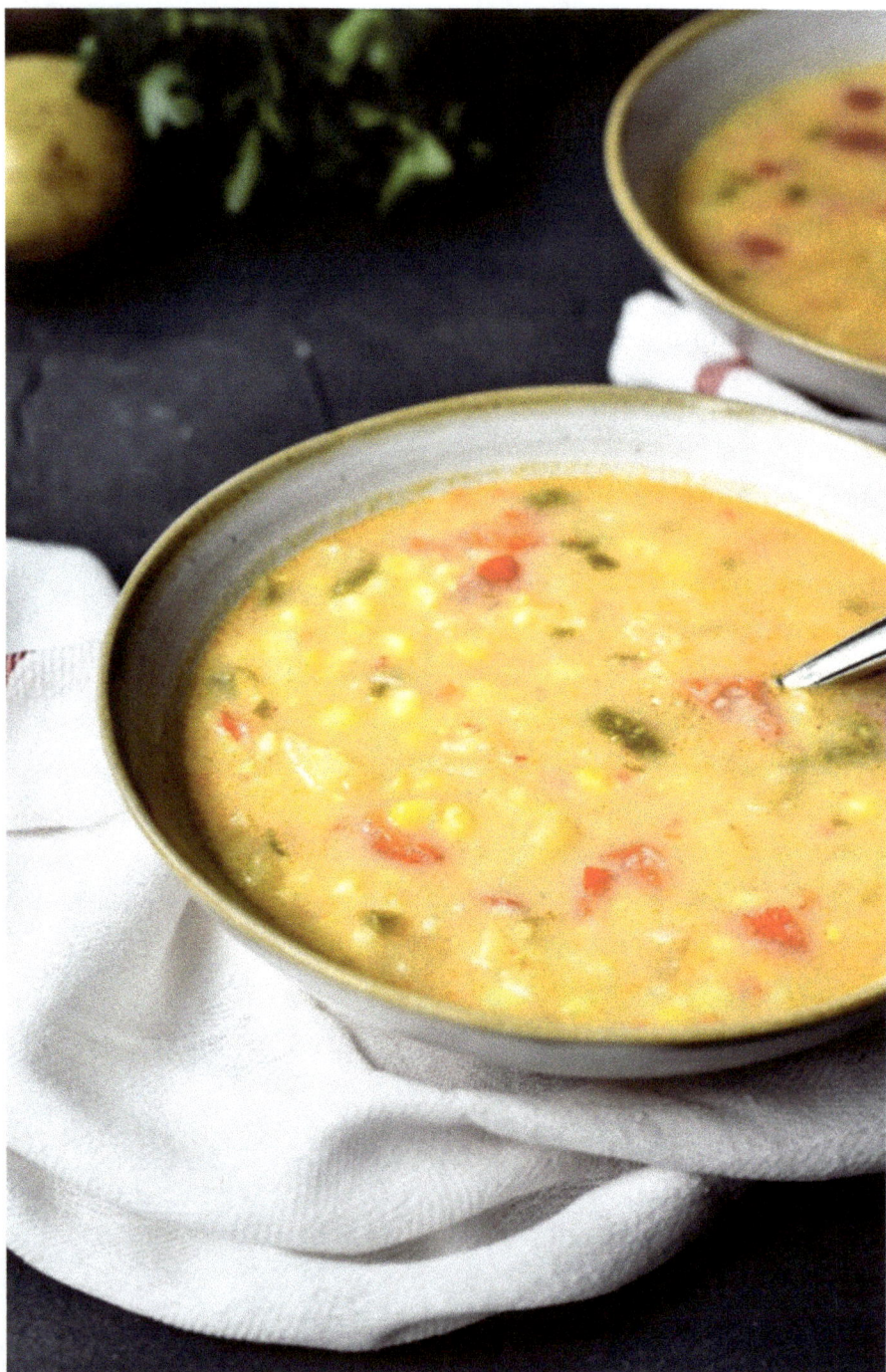

4-WEEK MEAL PLAN

Week 1

Monday
Breakfast: Tofu Frittata
Lunch: Pork Chops In Beer
Dinner: Stewed Tomatoes

Tuesday
Breakfast: Tapioca
Lunch: Creamy Beef Burgundy
Dinner: Oregano Salad

Wednesday
Breakfast: Fruit Oats
Lunch: Smothered Steak
Dinner: Black Beans With Corn Kernels

Thursday
Breakfast: Grapefruit Mix
Lunch: Pork For Sandwiches
Dinner: Stuffed Acorn Squash

Friday
Breakfast: Berry Yogurt
Lunch: Cranberry Pork Roast

Dinner: Greek Eggplant

Saturday
Breakfast: Soft Pudding
Lunch: Pan-asian Pot Roast
Dinner: Thyme Sweet Potatoes

Sunday
Breakfast: Black Beans Salad
Lunch: Short Ribs
Dinner: Barley Vegetable Soup

Week 2

Monday
Breakfast: Carrot Pudding
Lunch: French Dip
Dinner: Butter Corn

Tuesday
Breakfast: Apple Cake
Lunch: Italian Roast With Vegetables
Dinner: Orange Glazed Carrots

Wednesday
Breakfast: Almond Milk Barley Cereals
Lunch: Honey Mustard Ribs
Dinner: Cinnamon Acorn Squash

Thursday

Breakfast: Cashews Cake

Lunch: Pizza Casserole

Dinner: Glazed Root Vegetables

Friday

Breakfast: Artichoke Frittata

Lunch: Hawaiian Pork Roast

Dinner: Stir Fried Steak, Shiitake And Asparagus

Saturday

Breakfast: Mexican Eggs

Lunch: Apple Cranberry Pork Roast

Dinner: Cilantro Brussel Sprouts

Sunday

Breakfast: Stewed Peach

Lunch: Swiss Steak

Dinner: Italian Zucchini

Week 3

Monday

Breakfast: Lamb Cassoule t

Lunch: Glazed Pork Roast

Dinner: Cilantro Parsnip Chunks

Tuesday

Breakfast: Fruited Tapioca

Lunch: Swiss Steak In Wine Sauce

Dinner: Corn Casserole

Wednesday

Breakfast: Baby Spinach Shrimp Salad

Lunch: Italian Pork Chops

Dinner: Pilaf With Bella Mushrooms

Thursday

Breakfast: Coconut And Fruit Cake

Lunch: Italian Pot Roast

Dinner: Italian Style Yellow Squash

Friday

Breakfast: Apple And Squash Bowls

Lunch: Beef With Horseradish Sauce

Dinner: Stevia Peas With Marjoram

Saturday

Breakfast: Slow Cooker Chocolate Cake

Lunch: Oriental Pot Roast

Dinner: Broccoli Rice Casserole

Sunday

Breakfast: Fish Omelet

Lunch: Barbecued Ribs

Dinner: Italians Style Mushroom Mix

Week 4

Monday
Breakfast: Brown Cake
Lunch: Ham And Scalloped Pota toes
Dinner: Broccoli Casserole

Tuesday
Breakfast: Stevia And Walnuts Cut Oats
Lunch: Pork And Pineapple Roast

Wednesday
Breakfast: Walnut And Cinnamon Oatmeal
Lunch: Barbecued Brisket
Dinner: Dinner: Slow Cooker Lasagna

Thursday
Breakfast: Tender Rosemary Sweet Potatoes
Lunch: Barbecued Short Ribs
Dinner: Brussels Sprouts Casserole

Friday
Breakfast: Orange And Maple Syrup Quinoa
Lunch: Beer-braised Short Ribs
Dinner: Pasta And Mushrooms

Saturday
Breakfast: Vanilla And Nutmeg Oatmeal

Lunch: Lamb Stew

Dinner: Onion Cabbage

Sunday

Breakfast: Pecans Cake

Lunch: Barbecued Ham

Dinner: Cheese Broccoli

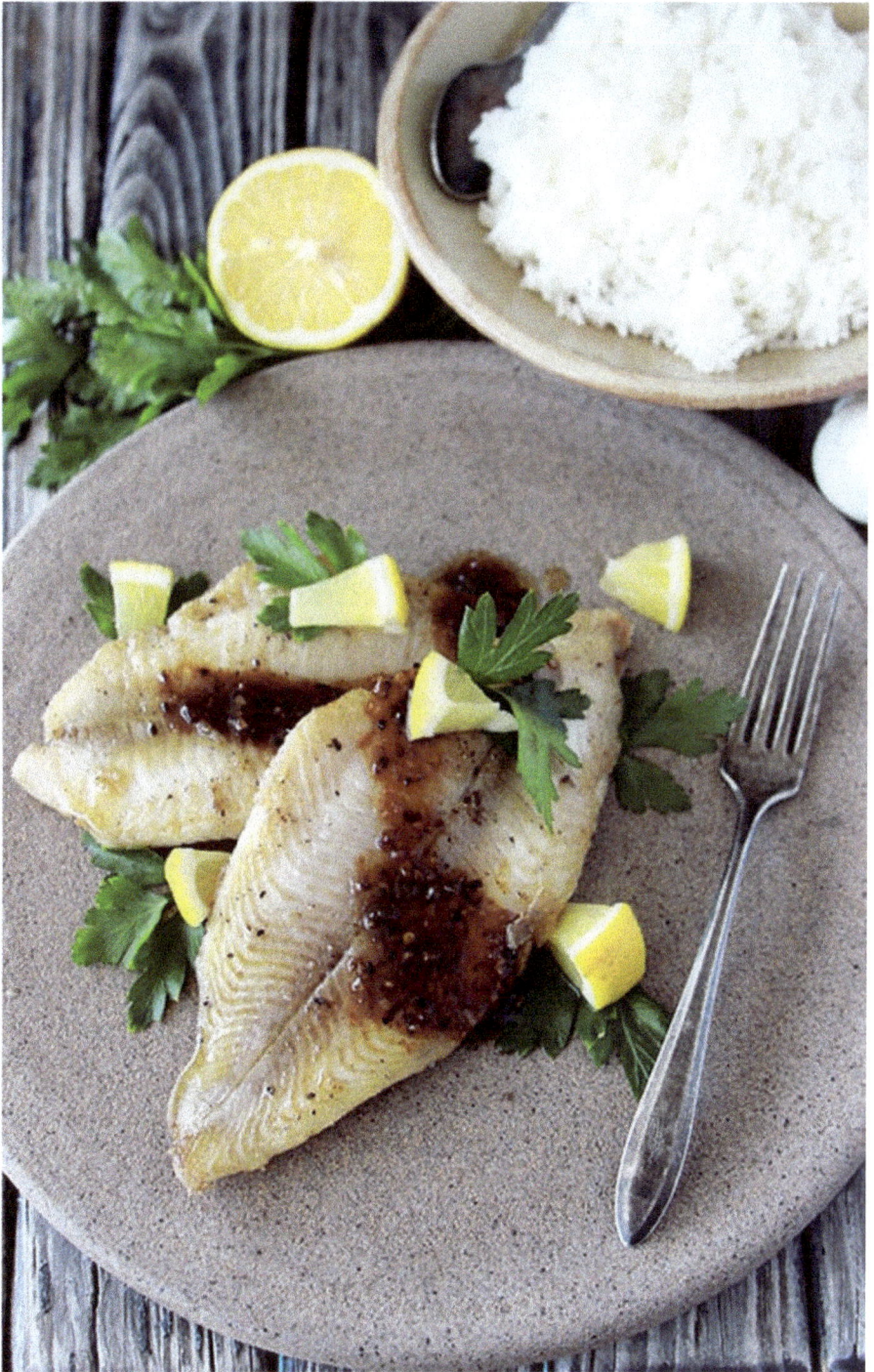

www.ingramcontent.com/pod-product-compliance
Lightning Source LLC
Chambersburg PA
CBHW050751030426
42336CB00012B/1757